Cambridge Elements ≡

Elements of Improving Quality and Safety in Healthcare
edited by
Mary Dixon-Woods,* Katrina Brown,* Sonja Marjanovic,†
Tom Ling,† Ellen Perry,* Graham Martin,* Gemma Petley,* and
Claire Dipple*
*THIS Institute (The Healthcare Improvement Studies Institute)
†RAND Europe

VALUES AND ETHICS

Alan Cribb,[1] Vikki Entwistle,[2] and Polly Mitchell[1]

[1]Centre for Public Policy Research, King's College London
[2]Health Services Research Unit, University of Aberdeen

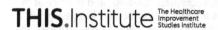

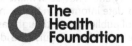

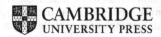

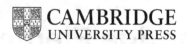

Shaftesbury Road, Cambridge CB2 8EA, United Kingdom

One Liberty Plaza, 20th Floor, New York, NY 10006, USA

477 Williamstown Road, Port Melbourne, VIC 3207, Australia

314–321, 3rd Floor, Plot 3, Splendor Forum, Jasola District Centre, New Delhi – 110025, India

103 Penang Road, #05–06/07, Visioncrest Commercial, Singapore 238467

Cambridge University Press is part of Cambridge University Press & Assessment, a department of the University of Cambridge.

We share the University's mission to contribute to society through the pursuit of education, learning and research at the highest international levels of excellence.

www.cambridge.org
Information on this title: www.cambridge.org/9781009325202

DOI: 10.1017/9781009325233

First published 2024

A catalogue record for this publication is available from the British Library.

ISBN 978-1-009-32520-2 Paperback
ISSN 2754-2912 (online)
ISSN 2754-2904 (print)

Values and Ethics

Elements of Improving Quality and Safety in Healthcare

DOI: 10.1017/9781009325233
First published online: April 2024

Alan Cribb,[1] Vikki Entwistle,[2] and Polly Mitchell[1]
[1]Centre for Public Policy Research, King's College London
[2]Health Services Research Unit, University of Aberdeen

Author for correspondence: Alan Cribb, alan.cribb@kcl.ac.uk

Abstract: Ethics involves examining values and identifying what is good, right, and justified – and why. Diverse values and ethical issues run through healthcare improvement, but they are not always recognised or given the attention they need. While much effort goes into understanding whether intervention X effectively leads to change Y, questions such as 'is X ethically acceptable?', 'does Y count as an improvement?', 'should Y be prioritised?', and 'if so, why?' are sometimes neglected. This Element demonstrates the ethical considerations and rich array of values that inevitably underpin both the goals of healthcare improvement (what aspects of quality or what kinds of good are pursued) and how improvement work is undertaken. It outlines an agenda for improvement ethics with the aim of helping those involved in healthcare improvement to reflect on and discuss ethical aspects of their work more explicitly and rigorously. This title is also available as Open Access on Cambridge Core.

Keywords: ethics, values, implicit normativity, ethical analysis, improvement ethics

ISBNs: 9781009325202 (PB), 9781009325233 (OC)
ISSNs: 2754-2912 (online), 2754-2904 (print)

Contents

1 Introduction   1

2 Ethics and Healthcare Improvement   1

3 The Practical Challenges of Bringing Ethical Analysis to Healthcare Improvement   23

4 Conclusions   25

5 Further Reading   26

Contributors   28

References   31

1 Introduction

This Element invites careful reflection on the somewhat contradictory-sounding idea that efforts to improve healthcare are rarely unequivocally good. It suggests deliberate and rigorous attention to:

- the rich array of values that underpin both the goals of healthcare improvement and enactments of improvement approaches
- the value judgements, tensions, and trade-offs involved in decisions about which goals to prioritise and which approaches to adopt.

These considerations are the focus of what we call 'improvement ethics'. The Element aims to help the people involved in improvement activities to engage in improvement ethics by highlighting how different values are embedded and prioritised in healthcare improvement. We also hope to encourage ethics scholars to contribute to investigation in this field by outlining a substantive agenda for improvement ethics as a rich field of inquiry that is ripe for development.

In Section 2, we introduce ethics and explain why ethical questions are central to healthcare improvement. We consider why some of the important ethical issues that come up in healthcare improvement work are sometimes neglected, either remaining unspoken or being passed over too quickly, and we outline some of the frameworks that can be drawn on in ethical reasoning. Section 3 indicates how improvement ethics can be expanded and enriched. We encourage attention to ethical issues that can arise first in identifying the purposes of and priorities for improvement (i.e. what counts as better healthcare and why?), and then in relation to improvement approaches and how improvement is pursued in practice. The section concludes with a set of starter questions to support explicit and broad-ranging reflection and debate about ethical aspects of improvement work. Section 4 offers some critical reflections on the challenges of bringing ethical analysis into healthcare improvement, acknowledging that ethical analysis is not easy and resolving many tensions is not straightforward. Despite these challenges, we suggest that active scrutiny of the values embodied in improvement work is as essential for rigour as scrutiny of evidence of effectiveness. Improvement ethics can and should be included as an integral part of healthcare improvement policy, practice, and research.

2 Ethics and Healthcare Improvement

2.1 Why Ethics Is Central to Healthcare Improvement

Ethics is a richly diverse activity that involves identifying and thinking about values and value judgements, and reasoning about what is good, right, and justified – and why. Ethical analysis includes a broad range of considerations, including whether, in what respects, and to what extent we (or others) are:

- treating people in acceptable ways
- bringing about as much good as we can
- working in ways that embody 'virtues' (ideal or valuable character traits or qualities)
- supported by social structures and cultures that foster these good actions and virtues.

Ethics is relevant to all aspects of human social life and activity, including healthcare, and is central to questions of improvement in this domain. Healthcare aims to bring about states that people value (including health) using processes that people value (including care). Claims about improvement are typically claims about what counts as good or better. In addition to the many different aspects of health and care that might be considered relevant to these claims, people pursuing improvements often apply a range of values associated with healthcare quality, including effectiveness, safety, patient-centredness, efficiency, equity, and timeliness. They also routinely make (or act in ways that reflect) value judgements about which aspects of quality or good healthcare should be prioritised and how best they should be addressed. Improvement processes and practices also incorporate values and enact value judgements, so people who make decisions about different improvement approaches or methodologies at least implicitly give different weight to considerations such as measurement validity and reliability, and attention and responsiveness to different stakeholders' perspectives.

One way of summing up the relationship between healthcare improvement and ethics is to say that healthcare improvement relies on ideas about what counts as good and better, and that ethical analysis involves the deliberate and sustained interrogation of those ideas. Ethical interrogation can consider which elements or aspects of good and better the ideas deployed in healthcare improvement include, what they miss out, and how (and how well) the different elements or aspects are interpreted and either combined or balanced together. Ethics can also usefully investigate, for example, what is good and right (or not), and why, in relation to how decisions are reached about priorities for improvement, and how improvement projects are approached.[1,2]

2.2 Implicit Normativity in Healthcare Improvement

The diverse values and ethical issues that are at play in healthcare improvement are rarely considered explicitly or in detail. There are at least two possible reasons for this. First, it might be assumed that people who work in healthcare should always be striving to make it better (or at least to ensure it is good enough), and that improvement work is inevitably good. With a little reflection, it is easy to see that improvement activities can have downsides (including unwanted side effects), that motivations for engaging in them can be mixed, and that their benefits and burdens may be unevenly distributed. These possibilities are not always rigorously considered.

Second, the main way in which improvement ethics has been discussed to date is in the context of the governance of improvement projects, and this focus may obscure important dimensions of improvement ethics. A key concern in debates about the ethical governance of improvement work has been to find a way to recognise and manage the ethical risks of improvement activities without blocking improvement progress.[3-6] Much attention has focused on the similarities and differences between improvement projects and research projects, and the development of guidance suitable for regulation and governance requirements.[7-11] Some important considerations have been identified and addressed, but this association with research ethics and governance has arguably constrained the scope of improvement ethics. In particular, the association may have led to the consideration of a narrower range of ethical concerns than are relevant to understanding and evaluating the goals of and approaches used in improvement practices.

The value judgements and ethical issues that are inherent in formulating healthcare improvement goals and selecting healthcare improvement approaches often remain unspoken and unexamined. Although improvement, by definition, aims to make something better, questions about what is good, right, or required, and therefore what would be better, are rarely brought to the surface – especially when widely accepted quality concepts such as effectiveness and safety are invoked. This phenomenon is sometimes called 'implicit normativity',[12] which has been defined as '... the presence of unstated or taken-for-granted assumptions about what is good and bad, right or wrong, required or not required'.[13] Implicit normativity is widespread in healthcare improvement. To some extent, this might be inevitable, but it is important to recognise that it can also lead to the neglect of important concerns or values.

To illustrate the point, we can consider a well-intentioned effort at increasing service efficiency. Imagine that the managers of a community nursing service are concerned about coping with rising levels of demand for their service and looking for ways to minimise wastage of staff time as they do so. They systematically redesign their staff deployment, journey routing, and timetabling to reduce staff travelling times and fit more visits to patients into each working week. Imagine their efforts achieve these goals. This could be claimed as an improvement in efficiency and perhaps enable the service to meet performance targets. But it also has the potential to indirectly diminish other aspects of the service that some patients and nursing staff may value highly. For example, relational continuity (the ongoing relationship between a patient and caregiver) might be reduced, and the service might become less responsive to people who have more time-sensitive needs. The pursuit of the worthwhile end of reducing waste could therefore have a negative impact on aspects of patient-centredness, effectiveness, and equity. The efficiency initiative might also come to shape how nursing staff routinely think and feel about their duties and priorities, and both nursing staff and managers could, on reflection, come to regret this. Over time, managers might start to re-examine the way they interpreted and prioritised the idea of service efficiency in relation to other important improvement ends.

Of course, improvement efforts are not always so narrowly focused, nor do they all diminish the perspectives of healthcare staff and patients in the way that happens in this example. From the outset, people seeking to improve healthcare are often conscious of navigating trade-offs between different aspects of quality or kinds of improvement, and some already engage in and encourage explicit deliberation about what matters most and why. As we will consider further below, some features of healthcare improvement methodologies can also help ensure that important ethical considerations, including different perspectives on what matters, are not overlooked. This example highlights the importance of recognising the phenomenon of implicit normativity in improvement efforts and of engaging in ethical reflection. This includes, when attempting to provide an ethical justification for improvement activities, thinking carefully and talking explicitly about the values that guide, and the various values that may be affected by, what is proposed.

Improvement ethics can involve, among other things, being alert to and analysing the often unspoken interpretation of good and the enactment of right in healthcare improvement goals and approaches.[1,2] Promoting professional reflection on the values and ethics embedded in healthcare improvement practices is one of our main concerns in this Element. Before concentrating on that theme – and to summarise other starting points that readers may be familiar with – we will first say something about some models and theories that are often drawn on in healthcare ethics (Section 2.3).

2.3 Theoretical Resources to Support Ethical Reasoning

When introducing ethics in Section 2.1, we noted that ethics is a richly diverse activity that involves consideration of a broad range of questions. Ethical analysis is not simple, and disagreements are likely. Answering questions about whether we're treating people in acceptable ways, bringing about as much good as we can, embodying virtues, and so on requires interpretation and value judgement. There is more than one way of determining what's acceptable, more than one interpretation of what it means to do good. It follows that it's not easy to answer ethical questions well. But as we have argued, questions of ethics are central to healthcare improvement, and there are at least two reasons why it's important to approach ethical issues explicitly and rigorously. First, it increases the chance that we will have at least taken into account the range of relevant considerations. Second, doing so puts us in a position where we can share the processes of reasoning that we have followed in coming to any conclusion, which enables scrutiny by and accountability to others.

Various theoretical resources have been developed to enable and support ethical reasoning. One rough guide to ethical reasoning that healthcare professionals are often taught about is the so-called 'four principles approach'.[14] This approach attempts to distil ideas from several different approaches to ethical reasoning (see summary in Box 1). The four principles can be understood as inviting us to consider four key questions:

- How and how far might possible actions produce benefits (considerations associated with the principle of *beneficence*)?
- How and how far can harm be avoided (*non-maleficence*)?
- Whether and how proposed actions treat people and their choices and values with respect (respect for *autonomy*)?
- Whether and how proposed actions treat different people fairly (*justice*)?

Many people find this simple framework helpful: the four principles are good general pointers, and the questions can stimulate productive thinking. However, despite its value as an introduction to ethical reasoning, the four principles framework is limited as a basis for ethical analysis and a guide for action. Each principle can be interpreted in multiple ways, and tensions between the principles will often arise when evaluating specific courses of action. In addition, some important ethical considerations (e.g. relating to solidarity and trust) are not easily analysed by just using the four specified principles.

Other theoretical resources (and often rich combinations of these) are used within the academic field of ethics. These resources enable debate about the nature and foundations of ethics and can also help inform ethical analysis. Due to differences in what they emphasise, different ethical approaches may be better suited to answering various ethical questions – but again, they are not simple-to-apply formulas and do not provide easy answers. Nevertheless, for those who have the opportunity and interest to engage with them, these resources can help

Box 1 Some influential approaches to ethical analysis – a very brief summary

Consequentialism: judges the rightness of acts according to their consequences.

Utilitarianism: a form of consequentialism that judges the rightness of acts according to the overall amount of *utility* (variously interpreted as happiness, preference satisfaction, or well-being) they bring about in a population.

Duty-based approaches: judge the rightness of actions according to their conformity with prescribed obligations or principles of right conduct. The obligations or principles may derive from a variety of sources, including religious and legal norms, human rights frameworks, and philosophical reasoning.

Virtue ethics: focuses on the characteristics of good people, attending to the ways virtuous people typically behave in different circumstances.

Feminist approaches: seek to make explicit and address gender-based injustices and other forms of oppression, including within other approaches to ethical analysis. These approaches typically encourage attention to the perspectives of people who are socially marginalised and disempowered.

Case-based approaches: consider how new or ethically unresolved cases compare and relate to other relevantly similar concrete examples that are ethically clear-cut. This may involve moving between several similar cases and comparing and contrasting them in order to make progress on understanding the new case.

clarify, extend, and strengthen accounts of ethical reasoning in particular situations. We can't do justice to the full range of approaches in this Element, but in Section 2.7, we offer a framework for stimulating thinking about improvement ethics in the form of questions for prompting reflection and discussion.

2.4 Extending Explicit Thinking about Ethics in Healthcare Improvement

In this section, we emphasise and further illustrate the need to move from implicit to explicit thinking about ethics in healthcare improvement. We can draw support for this idea from Don Berwick, an international expert in healthcare improvement. In a conference address, Berwick noted that, by the end of their careers, two founding figures of the healthcare quality movement had both come to see improvement work as rooted in ethical as well as technical concerns. He quoted Avedis Donabedian as saying, 'Ultimately the secret of quality is love' and W. Edwards Deming as saying, 'All that anyone asks for is a chance to work with pride'.[15] Berwick's address was wide-ranging, but the key point for us here is that while healthcare improvement leaders may not always have talked explicitly about values and value judgements, at least some of them have recognised that quality and ethics are intertwined.

2.5 Ethical Issues in Considering What to Improve

Paying explicit attention to purpose and priorities is important for critically considering justifications for healthcare improvement work.[7] The ethical justification of improvement efforts requires scrutinising our ideas about what is good in healthcare. Asking whether a change is an improvement should involve looking critically at:

- how it is characterised
- what it might be compared to and contrasted with
- why it is important.

Discussions about what is good in healthcare often refer to lists of dimensions of healthcare quality, such as the Institute of Medicine's widely known list of safety, effectiveness, patient-centredness, timeliness, efficiency, and equity.[16] These lists summarise features that are thought to deserve particular attention in improvement work and are sometimes considered to be the most important features of good healthcare systems and services. However, several aspects of their construction and some of the ways they are used in practice have ethical implications that are worth bearing in mind.

First, the items on the list represent a subset of a much wider range of values that people might believe are important when considering what matters for good healthcare.[2] If improvement initiatives are strongly oriented towards the listed dimensions of quality, then other aspects of healthcare may be neglected. For example, if funding schemes for improvement initiatives require applicants to indicate which of the listed dimensions of quality the work they propose addresses, other aspects will typically receive less attention. The items on a widely used list will sometimes be more justifiable as priorities for some healthcare systems or services than others. This will depend on the extent to which they reflect currently significant shortfalls and the priority concerns of the often diverse people who have a stake in particular systems or services. These people may include patients, employees or volunteers, and neighbourhood residents.

Second, the ways in which each item on a list is interpreted and specified – in particular, how they are operationalised into measures for assessing quality (or improvement) – also have ethical implications, including for which (and whose) needs and interests are prioritised. We saw this in the example of the community nursing service discussed in Section 2.2, which highlighted how a model of efficiency that focused on some inputs and outputs could obscure a number of other considerations of value that could be relevant both for efficiency and for quality more generally. Similar concerns arise for other quality concepts: for example, when effectiveness is specified and operationalised in narrow biomedical terms where a broader and diffuse set of consequences for health and well-being might be considered important. Also, when patient-centredness is assessed with a strong focus on patients' involvement in significant decisions about their care, shortfalls in respect, kindness, or continuity of relationships might be equally, if not more, important to patient-centredness in practice.[17]

Third, list presentations can be misleading in the way they present items as if they are similar kinds of things, equally important, and independent of each other.[18] As we also saw in the example in Section 2.2, the pursuit of improvement in one domain of quality (such as efficiency) will not always have positive or neutral implications for others. Often, there will be ethically significant trade-offs to be made. The apparent simplicity of lists should not be allowed to obscure the complexity of the value sets that need to be considered when justifying improvement interventions.

Sometimes, some rationale *is* given for an intervention in terms of how it makes things better, but the issues are not examined with enough depth or clarity. Just because something *works* in a narrow sense does not mean it is justified overall. Accordingly, scientific evidence for effectiveness in some respect will rarely be enough to justify an intervention. The fact that an intervention is effective in one way (towards a specified goal) should not be conflated with the idea that it is optimal or even right, all things considered. As Box 2 illustrates, questions of what would be good or better in healthcare often lead to a plurality of answers; all may be reasonable while none are necessary or sufficient in all cases.[19]

When we pay attention to the range of 'goods' that can be pursued or undermined by healthcare, we may conclude that some improvement interventions are not justified. A lot depends on the detail. Asking rigorous questions about a proposed intervention can reflect and enhance sensitivity to the complexities. We should be ready to reject what appear to be plausible or well-intentioned interventions after asking questions about: the strength of their evidence base; whether we can defend our account of what is good about them; and whether we have thought carefully enough about the harms they might embody or produce.

Box 2 Indicators of success suggested by healthcare professionals for their approaches to support people with long-term conditions

- ∘ Biomedical markers
- ∘ Symptom control
- ∘ Ability to perform particular functions (e.g. climb stairs)
- ∘ Psychological well-being
- ∘ General health and happiness
- ∘ Avoidance of undue treatment burden
- ∘ Ability to manage their condition in daily life
- ∘ Patient contributing to problem-solving and goal-setting
- ∘ Patient not being unduly dependent on formal healthcare services
- ∘ Open and effective communication between patient and healthcare professionals
- ∘ Accessibility of healthcare
- ∘ Communicating and relating in ways that are experienced as supportive

Adapted from Owens et al.[19]

However, an argument for rejecting or postponing an intervention is not the same as an argument for not intervening at all to address a shortcoming, and so there will always be an obligation to think about how to address it. This may involve exploring other interventions or thinking about how to refine and trial the proposed intervention. But any subsequent intervention should be accompanied by careful and self-critical evaluation to mitigate against ethical misgivings. Attending to the complexity of deciding what counts as an improvement doesn't justify blanket inertia or inaction; rather, it requires more broad-ranging and careful thought.

2.6 Ethical Issues in Different Approaches to Healthcare Improvement

We now turn to the values that are given more or less emphasis by particular approaches to improvement and examine some ethical aspects of the practical and methodological choices involved in these approaches. It's important to recognise the (often implicit) normativity in the development, selection, and advocacy of particular approaches to improvement, including what they designate and prioritise as improvement activities, what roles they establish, and who they present as relevant actors and stakeholders. Approaches to improvement are not ethically neutral, nor are they ethically equivalent. Each approach emphasises some specific values; each approach challenges those working on improvement to adhere to associated ideals and standards. At the same time, each approach also gives less prominence to (and can risk relative neglect of) some other values.

We use three broad improvement approaches – the Institute for Healthcare Improvement's Model for Improvement, collaboration-based approaches, and co-productive and co-design approaches – to illustrate some different value emphases and to highlight some of the ethical considerations that people working on improvement need to be aware of. In selecting these examples from the mainstream improvement literature, we acknowledge that we are relying on a relatively restricted idea of *an improvement approach*. Of course, a far broader range of activities and processes can contribute to healthcare improvement, including social movements and political activism, changes to funding patterns or professional preparation, and technological developments – but they are not the focus of this discussion.

These three approaches are featured and critically reviewed in the Elements on the Institute for Healthcare Improvement approach,[20] collaboration-based approaches,[21] and co-producing and co-designing,[22] respectively. The brief descriptions here are intended to enable us to highlight issues of values and ethics – some of which are also considered in the respective Elements. Our main contention is that the value emphases reflected in the different improvement approaches are not usually highlighted or debated enough. We suggest that much is to be gained in improvement ethics by drawing out the different value emphases associated with different approaches and looking across the full range of relevant values, including those that are given less emphasis when the focus is elsewhere. We stress that a similar analysis could be produced using a different sample of approaches.

In the following sections, we use:

- the Model for Improvement approach to introduce a cluster of ideas that might be denoted as practical-technical values associated with objective setting and measurement
- collaboration-based approaches to draw attention to the social values associated with collegial learning
- co-productive and co-design approaches to discuss the social values associated with inclusion and democracy.

As we will illustrate, each set of values is important, and they are not mutually exclusive. Each of the three improvement approaches positively emphasises some particular values and, as a result, can make some ethical challenges (including enacting those values and tensions between certain combinations of values) particularly evident. However, similar ethical challenges can also occur in other approaches. No improvement approach can be implemented without potential ethical pitfalls.

We note that our discussion of these approaches is deliberately broad and serves mainly to illustrate the different value dimensions that can be in play. More detailed improvement ethics analyses would need to look carefully at *how* different approaches are applied (and likely combined) in specific contexts.

2.6.1 Model for Improvement: The Importance of Practical-Technical Values

The Model for Improvement is among the best-known frameworks for approaching healthcare quality improvement.[23,24] As described by the Institute for Healthcare Improvement, it has two components. The first is a set of questions that are intended to help clarify the goals of an improvement effort, the changes that can be made to achieve those goals, and the measurements that might provide evidence of progress towards the goals.

- ○ What are we trying to accomplish?
- ○ How will we know that a change is an improvement?
- ○ What change can we make that will result in an improvement?

The second component is the testing and refinement of change, which takes place through plan-do-study-act (PDSA) cycles, supported by measurement strategies and techniques such as statistical process control charts (see the Element on statistical process control[25]). This two-part core provides a very general structure for thinking about and doing improvement work, so the model can be applied in diverse settings to an apparently limitless range of quality concerns.

The Model for Improvement exemplifies a number of features at the heart of the quality improvement tradition: it stresses the importance of being explicit and systematic in defining and refining aims, methods, and progress, and it emphasises the importance of accurate and repeated measurement of change in response to intervention. These features lead us to characterise the framework as one that foregrounds practical-technical values associated with objective setting and measurement. These practical-technical values are of substantial ethical importance. They can help people to provide justifications for their improvement goals, why the steps they are taking make sense, and how their progress can be demonstrated. But while having explicit and systematic goals and measurement may be necessary conditions of ethically defensible healthcare improvement, they are not sufficient conditions.

In practice, a strong emphasis on practical-technical values also carries ethical risks, and the significance of these risks depends on how carefully they are anticipated and managed. We will outline three examples here.

- First, an emphasis on technical standards for measurement might encourage a focus on improving aspects of healthcare that are easier to measure, but discourage efforts to tackle other important (perhaps less readily measurable) shortfalls, such as quality of communication (which is highly interpretive and subjective) or experiences of disrespect (which can occur in micro-communications and may be ambiguous or disputed).
- Second, people may tend to take numeric measures that are partial *indicators* of improvement too seriously and treat them as if they are perfectly valid or near-complete reflections of those aspects of quality (e.g. effectiveness) with which they are associated.[26] An emphasis on narrow indicators of success may obscure the bigger picture of what matters to people.
- Third, even if good progress is made in relation to specific objectives, the specification or measurement of those objectives may be too narrow. Side effects may go unseen if they are not predicted or otherwise not included in what is measured.[27]

In some respects, the Model for Improvement is especially well-placed to respond to these risks of what we might call 'technical closure'. As frameworks go, it's flexible, has been extensively debated, and has a history of refinements. The model also incorporates the idea of 'balancing measures', which encourages its users to employ a range of indicators that go beyond the core aims of their improvement intervention and to look outside their immediate objectives for potential side effects and complications.

But ethical issues can still arise in practice with applications of all improvement approaches, including the Model for Improvement. It's well understood within the field of quality and safety that no tool, model, or approach is self-applying: they all have to be applied by real people who work in diverse circumstances and are subject to a range of pressures and constraints. Ethical concerns can arise from the different ways in which the steps of a framework or approach are interpreted and implemented, and from the implications of these in particular circumstances. Here, we note three (perhaps overlapping) kinds of situations in which people may be particularly prone to being misled by technical thinking in improvement contexts.

- **A narrow focus or scope:** Narrowly circumscribed clinical improvement projects may be at particular risk of being misled by technical thinking because it is more plausible (and tempting) to have them rely too much on specific indicators, such as response times to the completion of clinically recommended actions or trends in key biomedical markers. When thinking about learning and improvement for healthcare systems, measurements need to be seen and interpreted in the context of a wider range of evaluative judgments (including those from patients' perspectives) and more holistic thinking.[28]

- **Activities informed only by a limited range of perspectives:** A small, relatively homogeneous group (e.g. of specialist healthcare practitioners) who decide and work in a top-down way to improve some aspect of healthcare may be particularly prone to thinking that their own priorities, interpretations, and favoured measures are adequate. A more diverse group could bring different and useful perspectives on the problem and proposed solution – but may at the same time introduce uncertainties and disagreements about what is better.[29]

- **Reliance on toolkit resources for the learning of improvement approaches:** The problems of narrow scope and limited perspective may be especially exacerbated when people learn about improvement approaches via toolkit-type resources and when they lack the experience or time to adequately consider cultural contexts and apply the necessary relational and 'soft' leadership skills for healthcare improvement.[20]

While the ethical risks of technical closure may be particularly severe for approaches that emphasise practical-technical values, they also apply to much other healthcare improvement work (using a variety of approaches) where the operational definition and measurement of success is a central concern. Although balancing measures are usually (and rightly) seen primarily as a counter to the risks of technical closure, the general idea behind these measures – that is, to moderate and integrate concern for specific indicators of improvement with more holistic thinking – also has broader implications. The need for holistic thinking goes well beyond considering specific goals and indicators or how benefits and harms are framed. For example, questions need to be asked about whether:

- actions introduced in pursuit of improvement disadvantage particular subgroups of patients
- there is enough transparency about what changes are being investigated
- patient and staff data are held securely and used in ways that people consider acceptable and that respect their interests.

We suggest that holistic thinking about these matters should be seen as a central strand of improvement ethics.

Attention to broader social values and more open-ended forms of reasoning can be incorporated *within* approaches such as the Model for Improvement when space is made for the kinds of situationally sensitive and compassionate insight and commitment associated with 'practical wisdom'.[30] As some leaders within the Institute for Healthcare Improvement have advocated, the model might also give serious attention to the perspectives of patients and people with relevant interests and insight who have often been marginalised from improvement work.[20,31] In Sections 2.6.2 and 2.6.3, we look briefly at approaches that are specifically designed with these considerations in mind: collaboration-based and co-producing and co-designing approaches.

2.6.2 Collaboration-Based Improvement Approaches: Promoting Collegiality and Shared Learning

Collaboration-based improvement refers to a family of network-based approaches, often involving work across institutions to develop, identify, and implement improvements.[21] Collaboration-based practices can be mapped on a spectrum: some examples of formally designated quality improvement collaboratives are highly organised, tightly topic-focused, and may follow a particular improvement model such as the Model for Improvement. Others, including many that are referred to as communities of practice, are loosely organised with relatively diffuse agendas and perhaps a less structured approach.[32]

The very word collaboration suggests a value-laden conception of improvement relationships. It brings to mind ideas of social relationships that have more of the mutuality associated with networks than the power disparities (and scope for exploitation) associated with hierarchies, or the competition (and scope for hostility) associated with markets. Networks can also be described in ways that clearly reflect certain values, as exemplified in this account which defines networks as '... cooperative structures where an interconnected group, or system, coalesces around shared purpose, and where members act as peers on the basis of reciprocity and exchange, based on trust, respect and mutuality'.[33]

The idea that collaboration and its associated values can enhance the effectiveness and efficiency of improvement activities is highly plausible. Collaboration between institutions and across geographical areas has the potential to harness people's energy and voluntary agency, support testing at scale, and enable learning through comparison. It may also reduce some of the hazards associated with managerial or marketised approaches – for example, top-down targets or relatively crude incentive structures that distort objectives and undermine, rather than reinforce, people's intrinsic or internal motivation for improvement. But the potential contribution to the effectiveness of improvement effort is not always evident[21] and is not the only reason to value collaboration-based approaches: advocates point to professional discourse (based on the knowledge, beliefs, and assumptions acquired through specialist training) that emphasises cooperative and friendly interaction, professional autonomy, and community-building – valuing these at least to some extent in their own right.

As with the Model for Improvement, a cluster of ethical issues can also arise in relation to collaboration-based approaches, and these can be relevant for other approaches too. There are questions of whether some collaboration-based improvement approaches are fit for purpose and live up to their values (see the Element on collaboration-based approaches[21]). For example, just calling something a collaborative does not mean it embodies all the values of collaboration: a group that has been designated a quality improvement collaborative (e.g. to help secure funding support) might, in practice, harbour uncooperative, competitive, or even hostile relationships.[34] This raises an important issue for improvement ethics more generally: they must be about more than the ethics of improvement interventions. Improvement interventions should not be seen as detached from the professional and social fields around them. This would be comparable to conceptualising clinical ethics as only about the ethics of particular treatment interventions and paying no attention to the importance of care relationships and what underpins them, such as the character, disposition, learning, well-being, or sustainability of the workforce.

Collaboration-based approaches remind us, then, that healthcare improvement involves 'context strengthening' – that is, fostering the conditions for collective learning and for *sustaining* (not just making) desirable changes to healthcare outcomes. Context strengthening involves taking a serious interest in the culture and relationships between people working on improvement activities and healthcare agents more generally. It raises ethical questions about how these can work well or go wrong, including by encouraging or discouraging professional virtues. This is not simply a point about precursors to or conditions for healthcare improvements in the form of clinical outcomes or rates of adoption of practices closely linked to these; rather, there is a need to recognise that healthcare cultures (including those fostered among people working on improvement) form part of healthcare and can, in themselves, be the difference between better or worse care. Improvement ethics needs to take into account matters of culture.

Although collaboration-based approaches to improvement often focus on identifying and spreading good practice in the form of appropriate treatments or care bundles for specific patient groups, the implications of their learning can be more extensive. Colleagues who have committed to working together for better health and who have significant social authority and influence could develop and pursue more expansive improvement ambitions, for example, to tackle challenges arising from the social and policy conditions in which health services operate and which can often be very influential on health outcomes.[15] Ethical and political questions become intertwined here, but questions of the scope and boundaries of professional responsibility are certainly important within improvement ethics.

The value-laden terms used to describe collaboration-based approaches imply that they are ethically good. There is a risk that some of those who adopt the terms to describe what they are doing are trading on this implication when their improvement efforts do not necessarily merit it. Improvement ethics needs to pay critical attention to which values are and are not reflected in practical enactments.

2.6.3 Co-Producing and Co-Designing: Pursuing Inclusion, Equality, and Democracy

The terms 'co-production' and 'co-design' are used inconsistently, but here we follow Glenn Robert et al. in using 'co-production' to 'recognise the two-way nature of services, that is, how the relationships and interactions between those providing and using a service influence the delivery, value, and outcomes of that service'. We use 'co-design' to refer to 'an intentionally applied process, used as a creative way of understanding experiences and improving services'.[22] Co-production is not necessarily an approach to improvement, but it is a means through which improvement interventions can be planned, implemented, and evaluated. For this reason, and because it has similarities with the co-design approach to improvement that are relevant to the ethical issues the two raise, we consider both here.

The notion of co-production and the approach of co-design both reflect a recognition that patients' perspectives often differ from those of healthcare professionals, and that those perspectives matter. Efforts to recognise and strengthen co-production, and the adoption of co-design, can also reflect concerns that healthcare – and healthcare improvement – should be more democratic and based on less hierarchical and somehow more equal relationships. The rationales for co-production and co-design approaches in improvement contexts are thus value-laden – and we might say they highlight patient-centredness and equity within improvement approaches. They also often include overtly ethical language,[35] but the activities to which the labels are applied do not always reflect the implied values.

The term co-production is sometimes used or understood as simply another way to refer to the patient and public involvement agenda, which is increasingly mainstream in many countries, including the UK. However, emphasising co-production can be part of attempts to redefine healthcare and improvement by reimagining mainstream involvement discussions. The ways in which people talk about patient and public involvement can indirectly reinforce the idea that health service organisations and professionals are central and in control, even as they invite (some) patients or members of the public to get involved and influence them.[36] By contrast, leading advocates of co-production seek to move beyond this to support more radically equal partnership working. Maren Batalden et al. define co-production as '. . . the interdependent work of users and professionals to design, create, develop, deliver, assess and improve the relationships and actions that contribute to the health of individuals and populations'.[37] Batalden et al. argue that approaches to healthcare improvement have been systematically misguided by the assumption that healthcare can be treated as a *product* that is delivered by some people to others, rather than as a *service* that is necessarily co-constructed. Once this is understood, they argue, it follows that the lenses through which improvement is conceived, conducted, and evaluated must be rooted in and combine multiple perspectives.

Co-design approaches to service improvement include methods for combining the contributions of patients and healthcare staff to shape both the formulation of improvement challenges and potential solutions.[28] Approaches such as experience-based co-design highlight the importance of people's lived experiences and also of designing and maintaining healthcare services that reflect the diversity of those experiences. As with collaboration-based improvement, it is possible to support co-design approaches on the basis of their practical contributions to valuable goals, but again, the evidence for this is limited[21] and, for these approaches, a key part of their rationale is that they can reframe what counts as valuable.

As with collaboration-based approaches, the fact that co-production and co-design have an explicit ethical dimension does not mean that they should be treated as ethically unproblematic, either in theory or application. Respectful working with patients and healthcare staff and attention to their perspectives are good, but they are not the only goods. Co-production and co-design thinking should encourage us to consider who has the opportunity and power to shape the ways in which healthcare is valued and improvement is undertaken, and who does not. They can also ask questions about the boundaries of improvement, not least to consider whether, when, and how far improvement ideas and activities can and should arise from outside the healthcare system, and who should be considered inside or outside.

A number of other questions and concerns that have been raised about co-production and co-design can also be understood as ethical issues.[22,37] These issues will be important areas of consideration for improvement ethics.

- Not all patients are equally willing and able to engage in co-production and co-design activities. The perspectives of some people, including those from ethnic minorities and with mental health diagnoses, may be vulnerable to being neglected in improvement work.[38,39] This raises concerns about equity and fairness in improvement processes as well as the adequacy of measured outcomes.
- Even when working in partnership is possible, it may be difficult to share accountability because healthcare professionals often have specific legal and moral responsibilities. Ethical questions may be raised about what's promised to improvement partners and how.
- More broadly, there can be tensions between patient and professional contributions that need to be managed. In some instances, there may be a risk of undervaluing professional expertise.
- An emphasis on being responsive to specific people and contexts may be in tension with some of the advantages of standardisation in healthcare service provision.

Again, these ethical challenges are not unique to co-production or co-design; they can arise in any type of improvement work that aspires to be responsive to patients' perspectives or to engage diverse participants and to do so in respectful ways.

The existence of ethical challenges and uncertainties is not an argument against co-production or co-design. One broader point that can be taken from this section is that ethical challenges are ever-present in improvement approaches, even when they are disguised or otherwise hidden from view. A key task of improvement ethics is to unmask the implicit normativity of approaches to, as well as the goals of, improvement and to bring ethical issues out into the open so that they can be more robustly considered and addressed.

2.7 Some Questions to Stimulate Ethical Reflection

In this section, we draw together some of the learning from earlier sections and offer a starter set of questions to encourage ethical reflection on improvement proposals and activities. People working to improve healthcare are probably already routinely asking some of these questions as they plan, develop, and reflect on their work. The questions in Table 1 are intended to help extend and deepen that reflection and discussion, making the implicit normativity of healthcare improvement work more explicit by further probing the ethical assumptions and implications of improvement work.

The set of questions does not exhaust those relevant to improvement ethics, and there is certainly scope to improve the set with learning that comes from experiences of using it. We suggest using the questions flexibly to open and

Table 1 A framework for organising questions to facilitate ethical reflection on healthcare improvement.

Questions to help characterise an improvement activity	Questions to support reflection on what makes healthcare good	Questions to support reflection on what makes improvement processes good and right
Which aspects of healthcare are intended to be improved, and in what respects? Why does the intended change amount to an improvement?	Whose vision of healthcare, and what sets of purposes, inform the identification of the problem and the aims of the intended improvement? Whose concerns might be less well reflected?	Are the processes for formulating aims, characterising and prioritising the problem and the improvement, and evaluating the improvement approach well justified?
• What harms, problems, or short-falls are identified and targeted for improvement?	• Why and for whom do the aspects of healthcare that are targeted for improvement matter?	• Are they respectful, fair, inclusive, and appropriately responsive to diversity?
• What kinds of benefits or improvements are anticipated from the proposed improvement activity?	• Does the intended improvement reflect lived experiences and what matters to people (not just biomedical or institutional concerns)?	• Do they arise from or enable collegial or broader collaborative or partnership working?
• What negative side effects might result from the intended improvement?	• Who experiences the main burden of the targeted problems, and who is most likely to benefit from the improvement? Who is less likely to benefit, and who might be adversely affected?	• What kinds of dialogues do they involve?
• What benefits might be lost by changing current practice?		• How are any divergences, tensions, or conflicts handled?

Table 1 (cont.)

Questions to help characterise an improvement activity	Questions to support reflection on what makes healthcare good	Questions to support reflection on what makes improvement processes good and right
	• What consideration or priority has been given to health inequalities? Does the intended improvement go beyond what is most readily measurable? Does it include more diffuse, qualitative considerations of what matters for good healthcare? What tensions arise in defining the success of the improvement activity? For example between: • different aspects of quality or different kinds of *better* in healthcare • the needs of and potential benefits to different groups of people • actions and effects at different levels in the healthcare system.	
What improvement interventions and approaches are being proposed, and why? Do they impose any new duties or responsibilities, and for whom?	Which health or social goods are (and are not) being pursued by and within the proposed interventions (and approaches)?	What value judgements are built into the methods and models used, the indicators or measures of improvement, and the construction of the evidence base? Whose perspectives and values are sought and

considered in:

- developing the intervention and approach
- selecting measures of improvement
- assessing and evaluating the improvement activity?

Who are the people working on improvement accountable to, and how?

Are established professional roles and identities changed?

Are the cultures of healthcare provision, and the virtues of healthcare practitioners, strengthened or undermined?

What scope is there, and how well is that scope used, to promote good (including more equal) relationships and ongoing sharing of learning?

Do they involve coercion or penalty for non-compliance?

Do they involve benefits or rewards for compliance?

Who shoulders the responsibilities, burdens, and costs of the interventions and approaches?

To whom do benefits accrue?

Is the implementation costly or resource intensive, and have these costs been factored into the overall assessment of its merits?

Are there any other concerns that something is not right about any aspects of the interventions or approaches being considered?

How are any uncertainties about answers to any of these questions dealt with?

help structure reflection and discussion. Questions are posed in the present tense, but they can also be asked prospectively (in the future tense) to guide planning and support justification of proposals or retrospectively (in the past tense) to support evaluative reflection and learning from experience. Some questions will be more relevant, and perhaps more readily answered, for some kinds of improvement work than others. Answers will, of course, depend on the particular improvement work being considered. People seeking improvement should also be prepared for the likelihood that others will answer some questions differently, even when they are thinking about the same improvement proposal or activity. Respectful consideration of why answers differ should enrich ethical understanding – and we include this within the scope of improvement ethics.

What constitutes the best ethical reasoning around any one question or set of questions may remain contested, and there may be several justifiable ways of moving forward despite this. Answers to the questions will not, in themselves, constitute a recipe for action, but they should help bring a range of relevant considerations out into the open. These considerations should allow for more deliberate, broad-ranging, and thorough analyses within improvement ethics, thus paving the way for the development of well-justified decisions.

We can briefly consider how some of these questions might be applied to a simplified scenario in Box 3.

Box 3 An initiative to improve access to an outpatient clinic

A virtual (digital) clinic system is designed and rolled out to underpin and extend effective access for quarterly check-ups for a group of outpatients. Plan-do-study-act cycles are used to achieve a high level of uptake and patient acceptability, as well as to improve the detection of complications and reduce the number of unplanned hospitalisations.

Answering the questions set out in Table 1 would, at least, require some familiarity with the way the current and proposed clinic systems work in context, and with the range of people involved. Social and moral awareness and imagination are likely to be useful, even if they only take us as far as identifying the further and more specific questions that warrant investigation. Conversation can be a very useful means of exchanging and expanding ideas about current situations, proposed interventions, and other possibilities – enhancing the range of questions asked and potential answers considered.[40] The initial responses to the digital clinic scenario in Box 4 are illustrative starters only.

> Box 4 Some questions to ask about the initiative to improve access to an outpatient clinic
>
> • What are the possible benefits related to health and well-being, and what are the risks and costs of the shift towards digital healthcare here? For example:
>   ○ Do some patients find the new arrangement better than the previous one? Which ones and why?
>   ○ Are some subpopulations newly or disproportionately disadvantaged by the digital shift? Which ones, how, and why?
>   ○ Can and should some level of existing outpatient facilities and services be preserved and deployed for those who will struggle with, or be disadvantaged by, the shift to a virtual (digital) service?
> • What are some of the more diffuse risks? For example:
>   ○ Are the same or equivalent professional peer support and educational opportunities available as those that arise from having a range of professionals and patients sharing the same physical space?
> • Do the improvement methods used neglect or obscure anything? For example:
>   ○ Should some different or additional measures of success be used, such as indicators of how well the virtual provision supports longer-term self-management?
>   ○ Was the patient population of the clinic involved in identifying the need for the virtual system and in designing the improvement? Did all staff have an opportunity to contribute meaningfully to the project? If not, might there be important concerns being missed?

This brief illustration shows that even with a broadly well-designed and successful initiative, it is important to self-consciously press home a broad range of questions about values and ethics. It is possible, in cases such as this, that *success* might hide significant failures, such as with regard to fairness or person-centredness.

3 The Practical Challenges of Bringing Ethical Analysis to Healthcare Improvement

We have been making the case that healthcare improvement is not a purely practical-technical activity and shouldn't be treated as such. Both the purposes of and approaches to healthcare improvement are inevitably underpinned by ethical values and reasoning, although often implicitly, and these need greater scrutiny. In this section, we consider some of the potential problems raised by our proposal that improvement ethics should feature clearly and prominently in improvement practice and research. Ethical analysis, as a process of careful scrutiny of the values that underpin the goals of improvement and pervade its practices, may seem liable to raise more problems than it solves. It's time-consuming, and it aims (some may say threatens) to bring previously unrecognised assumptions, ambiguities, and tensions to the surface. People who are working practically to improve healthcare may insist there is insufficient time or resources to resolve these issues adequately. If there is deep disagreement about values and priorities, ethical analysis may even threaten practical deadlock. We take these concerns seriously and address them briefly here.

First, we stress that ethical analysis should be thought of as integral to, rather than an obstacle to, considered and systematic healthcare improvement. Careful thinking about assumptions, implications, and consequences is central to the whole field of healthcare improvement, which already clearly recognises that simply saying that some intervention or approach is better than another does not make it so. Healthcare improvement seeks to show what does and does not work through systematic collection and analysis of evidence. Improvement ethics is broadly in harmony with this approach, as it seeks to carefully think through the ethical assumptions, implications, and consequences of improvement work.

Second, we agree that there is a need to strike a balance between thinking and doing. We are not proposing to turn people who work practically on healthcare improvement into armchair philosophers who spend so much time spelling out and grappling with all of the problems with improvement practice that they never get anything done. Taking ethics seriously does suggest exercising a certain amount of caution in decision-making, but it shouldn't result in being paralysed by the recognition that it's impossible to eliminate all disagreement, nor a dizzying sense that 'anything goes'. Indeed, not doing anything may be worse, ethically speaking, than doing something imperfect. Just as many decisions have to be made in the face of scientific uncertainty and scientific methods are open to criticism and modification, so decisions may have to be made in the face of some ethical contention and imperfections in the scope or processes of ethical analysis. Ethical reflection on the processes of ethical analysis should itself reduce the risk of excessive caution and failure to act.

We are not proposing that those seeking improvement need to do all the work of ethical analysis that might be envisaged. There is clear scope to further develop collaborations between people who work primarily on healthcare and its improvement and people who specialise in ethical analysis.[7] For example, ethics specialists might have particularly important roles to play in analysing and evaluating overviews of improvement work and in suggesting how careful ethical reflection can be fostered within curricula and cultures of improvement. The aspects of improvement ethics that we are encouraging people who specialise in healthcare and its improvement to carry out more routinely will mostly play out via deliberation, conversation, and reflection. Such deliberation would benefit from introductions to ethical reasoning, relevant examples of ethical analysis of improvement work, and question prompts of the kind provided in Table 1.

There can be a division of labour in improvement ethics. For example, individuals and project teams working on specific improvement initiatives need to focus on the ethical issues those initiatives raise and voice concerns when necessary. Those involved in thinking about improvement activities and practices at a collective level (e.g. at conferences or as part of collaboratives) need to think more generally about how they justify initiatives, including how they arrive at improvement priorities. And those in leadership positions (e.g. in policy development, healthcare services management, improvement activities, and research) need to think about the interactions between different initiatives, how to manage tensions between standardisation and diversity, and how to strengthen service cultures and contexts, including how to engage with system leaders and policymakers about priorities and questions of resource and governance. In all cases, ethical analysis involves standing back from practice and asking whether the values reflected in purposes and approaches are defensible. On occasions, and especially when looking more strategically at improvement priorities and system-wide agendas, it's important that the broad range of more or less overt norms that shape improvement activities are brought to the surface, considered together, and carefully debated. Opportunities for respectful conversation are likely to be key here.[40]

4 Conclusions

Improvement ethics should be seen as a key component of healthcare improvement, not just as an activity conducted by ethics specialists standing on the outside. Reflection on values and ethics should not be treated as supplementary to healthcare improvement; it's a core concern to be fully and explicitly integrated into the field.

Being critically attentive to values and ethics is part of rigour that's closely related to, and complementary to, attending to good-quality evidence to justify interventions. For healthcare practitioners and policymakers, it requires the willingness to discuss and debate the value commitments built into their work and the ethical issues these can give rise to. This might be a comparatively small adjustment for many individuals, but the implications are substantial for the field as a whole. Healthcare improvement discourses tend to be cast in largely scientific and technical terms. So, creating space for and giving prominence to debates about values and ethics requires both cultural change and practical effort. Evaluations of improvement work, too, need to expand both their conceptions of and engagements with ethics, perhaps particularly to engage with issues of inclusion and justice. There is a need to look beyond what is required for formal governance safeguards for specific projects to ethical questions that arise in all aspects of improvement work – from conception to enactment. This would mean those who study improvement embracing ethics as an allied field in the same way that they already embrace many other fields (e.g. social sciences, data science, and engineering). It means too, of course, that applied ethicists should consider adding healthcare improvement to their interests. Over time, it would make sense to bring together various strands of emerging work in improvement ethics to strengthen the area and further advance the kinds of debates reviewed in this Element.

5 Further Reading

General Introductions to Ethics

- Blackburn[41] – a very readable, general introduction.
- Beauchamp and Childress[14] – a classic text in medical ethics, which sets out four ethical principles for clinical decision-making.
- Peckham and Hann[42] – an edited collection introducing practical ethical challenges at the public health and health service levels.

Critical Insights into Ethical Aspects of Healthcare Improvement

- Aveling et al.[43] – a groundbreaking analysis, based on an ethnography of patient safety, on the interdependence of individual accountability and moral community in healthcare.
- Carter[13] – an insightful and clear account of implicit and explicit normativity in healthcare improvement.
- Cribb[7] – explores the value of a closer relationship between practically focused improvement science and more critical and normative improvement scholarship.
- Cribb et al.[1] – an argument for seeing narrower, more technical quality improvement lenses, including measurement, within broader, more open-ended conceptions of improvement and ethical evaluation.

○ Lynn et al.[6] – an important review of the ethics of quality improvement activities, comparing and contrasting them with healthcare research activities and arguing for a separate model of governance and accountability.

○ Mitchell et al.[2] – a pluralist account of healthcare quality, which argues that different conceptions of quality are appropriately invoked in different contexts, for different purposes.

Contributors

All the authors made a major contribution to the conceptualisation and drafting of the Element. Alan Cribb wrote an outline and the first draft, with contributions from Polly Mitchell. Vikki Entwistle significantly revised and extended the Element, and all authors contributed to subsequent edits. All authors have approved the final version.

Conflicts of Interest

None. This work was informed by our Wellcome Trust funded project, *'But why is that better?' An investigation of what applied philosophy and ethics can bring to quality improvement work in healthcare* [209811/Z/17/Z], which we are pleased to acknowledge.

Acknowledgements

We thank the peer reviewers for their insightful comments and recommendations to improve the Element. A list of peer reviewers is published at www.cambridge .org/IQ-peer-reviewers.

Funding

This Element was funded by THIS Institute (The Healthcare Improvement Studies Institute, www.thisinstitute.cam.ac.uk). THIS Institute is strengthening the evidence base for improving the quality and safety of healthcare. THIS Institute is supported by a grant to the University of Cambridge from the Health Foundation – an independent charity committed to bringing about better health and healthcare for people in the UK.

About the Authors

Alan Cribb is a professor of bioethics and education and Co-director of the Centre for Public Policy Research at King's College London. His research relates to applied philosophy and health policy. He has a particular interest in developing interdisciplinary scholarship that links philosophical, social science, and professional concerns.

Vikki Entwistle is a professor of health services research and philosophy at the University of Aberdeen. Her research and teaching are highly interdisciplinary. She uses philosophy and social research to understand and address concerns about quality, ethics, and social justice in healthcare, public health work, and funeral provision.

Polly Mitchell is a postdoctoral research fellow at King's College London. She worked for several years in healthcare quality improvement, managing a national clinical audit project, and researching patient-reported outcomes. Her research interests are varied, spanning moral and political philosophy, but chiefly relate to the philosophy of health and well-being.

Creative Commons License

References

1. Cribb A, Entwistle V, Mitchell P. What does 'quality' add? Towards an ethics of healthcare improvement. *J Med Ethics* 2020; 46: 118–22. https://doi.org/10.1136/medethics-2019-105635.

2. Mitchell P, Cribb A, Entwistle VA. Defining what is good: Pluralism and healthcare quality. *Kennedy Inst Ethics J* 2019; 29: 367–88. https://doi.org/10.1353/ken.2019.0030.

3. Jennings B, Baily MA, Bottrell M, Lynn J. *Health Care Quality Improvement: Ethical and Regulatory Issues.* Garrison, NY: The Hastings Center; 2007. www.thehastingscenter.org/wp-content/uploads/Health-Care-Quality-Improvement.pdf (accessed 2 February 2023).

4. Dixon N. *Guide to Managing Ethical Issues in Quality Improvement or Clinical Audit Projects.* London: Healthcare Quality Improvement Partnership; 2017. www.hqip.org.uk/wp-content/uploads/2017/02/guide-to-managing-ethical-issues-in-quality-improvement-or-clinical-audit-projects.pdf (accessed 2 February 2023).

5. Baily MA, Bottrell M, Lynn J, Jennings B. The ethics of using QI methods to improve health care quality and safety. *Hastings Cent Rep* 2006; 36: S1–40. https://doi.org/10.1353/hcr.2006.0054.

6. Lynn J, Baily MA, Bottrell M, et al. The ethics of using quality improvement methods in health care. *Ann Intern Med* 2007; 146: 666–73. https://doi.org/10.7326/0003-4819-146-9-200705010-00155.

7. Cribb A. Improvement science meets improvement scholarship: Reframing research for better healthcare. *Health Care Anal* 2018; 26: 109–23. https://doi.org/10.1007/s10728-017-0354-6.

8. Fiscella K, Tobin JN, Carroll JK, He H, Ogedegbe G. Ethical oversight in quality improvement and quality improvement research: New approaches to promote a learning health care system. *BMC Med Ethics* 2015; 16: 63. https://doi.org/10.1186/s12910-015-0056-2.

9. Faden RR, Kass NE, Goodman SN, et al. An ethics framework for a learning health care system: A departure from traditional research ethics and clinical ethics. *Hastings Cent Rep* 2013; 43: S16–27. https://doi.org/10.1002/hast.134.

10. Casarett D, Karlawish JH, Sugarman J. Determining when quality improvement initiatives should be considered research: Proposed criteria and potential implications. *JAMA* 2000; 283: 2275–80. https://doi.org/10.1001/jama.283.17.2275.

11. Nerenz DR, Stoltz PK, Jordan J. Quality improvement and the need for IRB review. *Qual Manag Health Care* 2003; 12: 159–70. https://doi.org/10.1097/00019514-200307000-00006.

12. Molewijk AC, Stiggelbout AM, Otten W, Dupuis HM, Kievit J. Implicit normativity in evidence-based medicine: A plea for integrated empirical ethics research. *Health Care Anal* 2003; 11: 69–92. https://doi.org/10.1023/A:1025390030467.

13. Carter SM. Valuing healthcare improvement: Implicit norms, explicit normativity, and human agency. *Health Care Anal* 2018; 26: 189–205. https://doi.org/10.1007/s10728-017-0350-x.

14. Beauchamp TL, Childress JF. *Principles of Biomedical Ethics, 8th ed.* New York: Oxford University Press; 2019.

15. Berwick D. Quality, Mercy, and the Moral Determinants of Health. Orlando, FL: Institute of Healthcare Improvement National Forum; 11 December 2019.

16. Institute of Medicine (US) Committee on Quality of Health Care in America. *Crossing the Quality Chasm: A New Health System for the 21st Century.* Washington, DC: National Academy Press; 2001. www.ncbi.nlm.nih.gov/books/NBK222274 (accessed 2 February 2023).

17. Entwistle V, Cribb A, Mitchell P, Walter S. Unifying and universalizing personalised care? An analysis of a national curriculum with implications for policy and education relating to person-centred care. *Patient Education and Counseling* 2022; 105: 3422–28. https://doi.org/10.1016/j.pec.2022.07.003.

18. Ledin P, Machin D. How lists, bullet points and tables recontextualize social practice: A multimodal study of management language in Swedish universities. *Critical Discourse Studies* 2015; 12: 463–81. https://doi.org/10.1080/17405904.2015.1039556.

19. Owens J, Entwistle VA, Cribb A, et al. 'Was that a success or not a success?': A qualitative study of health professionals' perspectives on support for people with long-term conditions. *BMC Fam Pract* 2017; 18: 39. https://doi.org/10.1186/s12875-017-0611-7.

20. Boaden R, Furnival J, Sharp C. The institute for healthcare improvement approach. In Dixon-Woods M, Brown K, Marjanovic S, et al., editors. *Elements of Improving Quality and Safety in Healthcare.* Cambridge: Cambridge University Press; forthcoming.

21. Martin G, Dixon-Woods M. Collaboration-based approaches. In Dixon-Woods M, Brown K, Marjanovic S, et al., editors. *Elements of Improving Quality and Safety in Healthcare.* Cambridge: Cambridge University Press; 2022. https://doi.org/10.1017/9781009236867.

22. Robert G, Locock L, Williams O, et al. Co-producing and Co-designing. In Dixon-Woods M, Brown K, Marjanovic S, et al., editors. *Elements of Improving Quality and Safety in Healthcare.* Cambridge: Cambridge University Press; 2022. https://doi.org/10.1017/9781009237024.

23. Langley GJ. *The Improvement Guide: A Practical Approach to Enhancing Organizational Performance, 2nd ed.* San Francisco, CA: Jossey-Bass; 2009.

24. Institute for Healthcare Improvement. How to improve. www.ihi.org/resources/Pages/HowtoImprove/default.aspx (accessed 4 December 2023).

25. Mohammed MA. Statistical process control. In Dixon-Woods M, Brown K, Marjanovic S, et al., editors. *Elements of Improving Quality and Safety in Healthcare.* Cambridge: Cambridge University Press; forthcoming.

26. Bevan G, Hood C. What's measured is what matters: Targets and gaming in the English public health care system. *Public Adm* 2006; 84: 517–38. https://doi.org/10.1111/j.1467-9299.2006.00600.x.

27. Pflueger D. Accounting for quality: On the relationship between accounting and quality improvement in healthcare. *BMC Health Serv Res* 2015; 15: 178. https://doi.org/10.1186/s12913-015-0769-4.

28. Dixon-Woods M, Martin GP. Does quality improvement improve quality? *Future Hosp J* 2016; 3: 191–4. https://doi.org/10.7861/futurehosp.3-3-191.

29. Donetto S, Pierri P, Tsianakas V, Robert G. Experience-based co-design and healthcare improvement: Realizing participatory design in the public sector. *Design J* 2015; 18: 227–48. https://doi.org/10.2752/175630615x14212498964312.

30. Dixon-Woods M. The problem of context in quality improvement. In Bamber RJ, editor. *Perspectives on Context: A Selection of Essays Considering the Role of Context in Successful Quality Improvement.* London: The Health Foundation; 2014: 87–99. www.health.org.uk/publications/perspectives-on-context.

31. Batalden P. Getting more health from healthcare: Quality improvement must acknowledge patient coproduction – an essay by Paul Batalden. *BMJ* 2018; 362: k3617. https://doi.org/10.1136/bmj.k3617.

32. de Silva D. *Improvement Collaboratives in Health Care.* London: The Health Foundation; 2014. www.health.org.uk/sites/default/files/ImprovementCollaborativesInHealthcare.pdf (accessed 2 February 2023).

33. Randall S. *Leading Networks in Healthcare.* London: The Health Foundation; 2013. www.health.org.uk/sites/default/files/LeadingNetworksInHealthcare.pdf (accessed 2 February 2023).

34. Carter P, Ozieranski P, McNicol S, Power M, Dixon-Woods M. How collaborative are quality improvement collaboratives: A qualitative study

in stroke care. *Implement Sci* 2014; 9: 32. https://doi.org/10.1186/1748-5908-9-32.

35. Williams O, Sarre S, Papoulias SC, et al. Lost in the shadows: Reflections on the dark side of co-production. *Health Res Policy Syst* 2020; 18: 43. https://doi.org/10.1186/s12961-020-00558-0.

36. Williams O, Robert G, Martin GP, Hanna E, O'Hara J. Is co-production just really good PPI? Making sense of patient and public involvement and co-production networks. In Bevir M, Waring J, editors. *Decentring Health and Care Networks*. Heidelberg: Palgrave Macmillan; 2020: 213–237.

37. Batalden M, Batalden P, Margolis P, et al. Coproduction of healthcare service. *BMJ Qual Saf* 2016; 25: 509–17. https://doi.org/10.1136/bmjqs-2015-004315.

38. Ocloo J, Matthews R. From tokenism to empowerment: Progressing patient and public involvement in healthcare improvement. *BMJ Qual Saf* 2016; 25: 626–32. https://doi.org/10.1136/bmjqs-2015-004839.

39. Gilbert D. *The Patient Revolution: How We Can Heal the Healthcare System*. London: Jessica Kingsley Publishers; 2020.

40. Cribb A, Entwistle V, Mitchell P. Talking it better: Conversations and normative complexity in healthcare improvement. *Med Hum* 2021; 48: 85–93.

41. Blackburn S. *Ethics: A Very Short Introduction*. Oxford: Oxford University Press; 2003.

42. Peckham S and Hann A. *Public Health Ethics and Practice*. Bristol: Policy Press; 2009.

43. Aveling EL, Parker M, Dixon-Woods M. What is the role of individual accountability in patient safety? A multi-site ethnographic study. *Soc Health Illness* 2016; 38: 216–32. https://doi.org/10.1111/1467-9566.12370.

Gemma Petley
THIS Institute (The Healthcare Improvement Studies Institute)

Gemma is Senior Communications and Editorial Manager at THIS Institute, responsible for overseeing the production and maximising the impact of the series.

Claire Dipple
THIS Institute (The Healthcare Improvement Studies Institute)

Claire is Editorial Project Manager at THIS Institute, responsible for editing and project managing the series.

About the Series

The past decade has seen enormous growth in both activity and research on improvement in healthcare. This series offers a comprehensive and authoritative set of overviews of the different improvement approaches available, exploring the thinking behind them, examining evidence for each approach, and identifying areas of debate.

Cambridge Elements ≡

Improving Quality and Safety in Healthcare

Elements in the Series

Collaboration-based Approaches
Graham Martin and Mary Dixon-Woods

Co-Producing and Co-Designing
Glenn Robert, Louise Locock, Oli Williams, Jocelyn Cornwell, Sara Donetto, and
Joanna Goodrich

The Positive Deviance Approach
Ruth Baxter and Rebecca Lawton

Implementation Science
Paul Wilson and Roman Kislov

Making Culture Change Happen
Russell Mannion

Operational Research Approaches
Martin Utley, Sonya Crowe, and Christina Pagel

Reducing Overuse
Caroline Cupit, Carolyn Tarrant, and Natalie Armstrong

Simulation as an Improvement Technique
Victoria Brazil, Eve Purdy, and Komal Bajaj

Workplace Conditions
Jill Maben, Jane Ball, and Amy C. Edmondson

Governance and Leadership
Naomi Fulop and Angus I. G. Ramsay

Health Economics
Andrew Street and Nils Gutacker

Approaches to Spread, Scale-Up, and Sustainability
Chrysanthi Papoutsi, Trisha Greenhalgh, and Sonja Marjanovic

Statistical Process Control
Mohammed Amin Almehmadi

Values and Ethics
Alan Cribb, Vikki Entwistle, and Polly Mitchell

A full series listing is available at: www.cambridge.org/IQ

Cambridge Elements ☰

Improving Quality and Safety in Healthcare

Elements in the Series

Collaboration-Based Approaches
Graham Martin and Mary Dixon-Woods

Co-Producing and Co-Designing
Glenn Robert, Louise Locock, Oli Williams, Jocelyn Cornwell, Sara Donetto, and
Joanna Goodrich

The Positive Deviance Approach
Ruth Baxter and Rebecca Lawton

Implementation Science
Paul Wilson and Roman Kislov

Making Culture Change Happen
Russell Mannion

Operational Research Approaches
Martin Utley, Sonya Crowe, and Christina Pagel

Reducing Overuse
Caroline Cupit, Carolyn Tarrant, and Natalie Armstrong

Simulation as an Improvement Technique
Victoria Brazil, Eve Purdy, and Komal Bajaj

Workplace Conditions
Jill Maben, Jane Ball, and Amy C. Edmondson

Governance and Leadership
Naomi J. Fulop and Angus I. G. Ramsay

Health Economics
Andrew Street and Nils Gutacker

Approaches to Spread, Scale-Up, and Sustainability
Chrysanthi Papoutsi, Trisha Greenhalgh, and Sonja Marjanovic

Statistical Process Control
Mohammed Amin Mohammed

Values and Ethics
Alan Cribb, Vikki Entwistle, and Polly Mitchell

A full series listing is available at: www.cambridge.org/IQ

Printed in the United States
by Baker & Taylor Publisher Services